GREEN EATING & PROTEIN
FOR LEANER ARMS

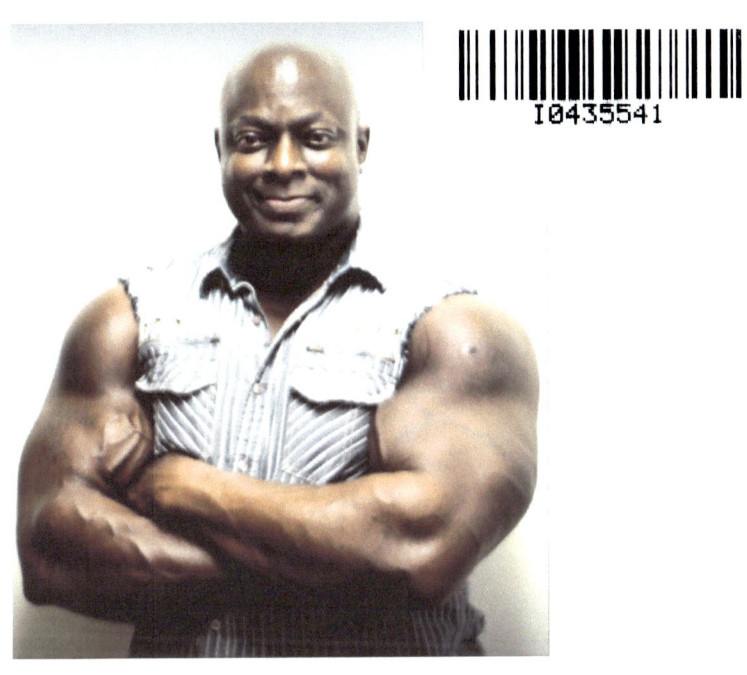

I0435541

Copyright © 2016 by Daryl Jones

Green Eating & Protein For Leaner Arms
By Daryl BIG"D" Jones

Green Eating & Protein For Leaner Arms is intended to be used for general guidelines only and no exercise of any kind, including those in this book, should be attempted without first consulting with a doctor and determining your physical suitability for strenuous exercise. The results in the book are not guaranteed and individual results will vary depending on many factors not addressed in this book.

Green Eating & Protein For Leaner Arms
By Daryl BIG"D" Jones

Table of Contents

Foreword

I was born an only child in Berkeley, California and raised by my single mom in Los Angeles. My mom worked hard to raise me as best she could and looking back I must say she did an awesome job as I wanted for nothing due to her many sacrifices for me.

Growing up in Los Angeles was tough, so in 1974 my mom decided to pack us up and move to the great northwest city of Portland, Oregon. I hated the move but at the ripe old age of 9 I had no say in the matter at all. Looking back, I realize that, like most parents, my mother knew best as we lived in an area that was calmer and more relaxed compared to Los Angeles. I understand now that not only did she take me to a much safer environment but she also basically saved my life, as I'm sure I would have become a complete product of my environment and went down the wrong path. Being in Portland also gave me male role models to follow in my family and the main one was my grandfather, Papa JJ. He was a man among men, tough when he needed to be but always very helpful and kind. What made the strongest impression on me was his endless love for his family. My grandfather was a man of dignity and deep family values. He instilled in me just how important it was to work hard at anything you do and to always exceed expectations. He got up at the same time every morning, work or no work, and you could set your clock to the squelching sound of the shower coming on at 3 AM every single day.

Green Eating & Protein For Leaner Arms
By Daryl BIG"D" Jones

This is probably why I say today that nothing comes to a sleeper except a dream. In order to make any dream a reality you have to get up and work towards it on a daily basis. The example that he and my uncles set for me has made me who I am today and I'm very thankful for that upbringing. It just seems natural now that I ended up pursuing a sport that takes work, sacrifice and self-discipline. I first began lifting weights when I was 14 years old in the summer of 1979. I was visiting my two cousins in Los Angeles after not seeing them for nine months. When I arrived at their house I right away realized that both Tommy and Tony had changed from the last time I saw them: they had developed serious biceps that I right away envied! I was curious how they did it and they both laughed and promised to show me later that day. The fact that Tommy continued to flex his biceps made my curiosity grow stronger by the minute. Finally, the evening came and they took me three houses down to their neighbor Michael's house and there in the backyard was a weight bench and some old weights, but to me those weights looked like a freshly baked chocolate cake to a fat kid left in a room all alone, except this chocolate cake could give me arms like my two cousins. I didn't know it at the time but this day would single-handedly change my entire life. I lifted weights with them that entire summer and when I returned to Portland the first thing I asked my mom was for my very own set of weights for Christmas.

Green Eating & Protein For Leaner Arms
By Daryl BIG"D" Jones

Once I started lifting weights I found it nearly impossible to stop, I couldn't imagine why everyone didn't want this awesome feeling that weight training gives you. At the age of 14 I knew that my mom was Santa and not some fat guy coming down the chimney (mainly because we didn't even have a chimney). When Christmas finally came around, I was elated when my mom gave me my very own 156-pound plastic-wrapped concrete weight set! I was one happy kid. We didn't have enough space for it in the living room of our two bedroom apartment, so I placed the weights at the foot of my bed and continued to train as I had in the summer of 79 (1979). I lifted those weights every day until I was able to bench press the entire 156 lbs. ten times without a spotter. I then felt I was ready to lift with the guys at school without being totally embarrassed. I was born with asthma, which prevented me from participating in a lot of physical activities and childhood sports. Too much running around would trigger my asthma and force me to sit and watch other kids play instead of participating. Even playing tag would cause me to become very ill with my asthma. During a visit to my doctor for a check-up, I shared with him that I had started training with weights. He advised me to continue doing it as it wouldn't aggravate my asthma and, in fact, might even be a good thing for me and help me to not overcome it but to possibly minimize the frequency of my asthma attacks.

As time went by I started to notice that my asthma attacks became less and less frequent.

Green Eating & Protein For Leaner Arms
By Daryl BIG"D" Jones

Now I can't scientifically prove that my weight training alone helped reduce my asthma, but I can say that I seemed to be able participate in more physical activities without it triggering an attack. So I continued to lift and gain confidence and feel more like a normal kid without any breathing issues. As time went on I began to realize that my life would never be the same again and I dreamed of someday becoming a professional bodybuilder. Weightlifting had caused a physical and mental transformation in me. Over the years, weight training has not only changed my outlook on life but has also opened up a host of opportunities such as being a personal trainer for important people, a bodyguard for different celebrities, and a Hollywood actor in movies and TV shows. I also competed in numerous bodybuilding competitions over the years and I can proudly say that in California I was fortunate to have won all my NPC (National Physique Committee) bodybuilding competitions, taking either first place in my weight class and/or winning the overall championship. I never got second place when I competed in the state of California, which seems amazing to me and as I look back this was a huge blessing as well. Lifting weights has definitely changed my entire life by giving me self-confidence and a positive mental attitude. It made me feel that I could accomplish anything I set my mind to. Weight training is, and always will be, my primary lifestyle. It has been so positive for me that I have made it my mission to share its benefits with the world.   *-Daryl "BIG D" Jones*

1. Introduction

Most men don't believe that women can accomplish the same fitness goals as they do. The truth is quite the opposite, in fact not only can women accomplish the same fitness goals, but the truth be told women (in my opinion) have a higher level of discipline, than "most" men. Now the reason I say these things are from my own personal observation over the past 36 years in the gyms across the country. Now about the only thing that women in the fitness world can't do the same as men is grow equally as large as a man.

For men or anyone else to think or believe that women can't accomplish similar goals such as developing their arms to become not only well defined and toned but also having the ability to increase the strength of their arms, is not only wrong but is also displaying a very shallow style of thinking. Now in the old days it was very common to believe that women can't do as men do in many areas of life, but as time has gone by this way of thinking has been proven to be incorrect.

Women have not only proven this way of thinking to be wrong time and time again, but over the years women have been allowed to more freely participate in such events as simply going in to a gym and lifting weights as men do. We have since seen countless women do the once thought to be impossible and now proven to be possible and this includes having stronger muscles. Not only have women now been doing this for quite some time but they have also taken those proven capabilities to even higher levels.

Green Eating & Protein For Leaner Arms
By Daryl BIG"D" Jones

Two women who are now known as the first "ever" women to become US Army Rangers, First Lt. Shaye Haver and Capt. Kristen Griest, on August 21st 2015 these two women accomplished the once thought to be physically as well as mentally impossible for any woman to ever successfully achieve, and that was to past a series of the most intense physically challenging test that the US armed forces has ever compiled to become a US Army Ranger. To fully understand the magnitude of this accomplishment, you'd have to understand that most men fail this goal during the first four days of RAP (Ranger Assessment Phase).

Now I mention these two women as they are not only the most recent to make American history, but they made history by breaking down another thought to be impossible physical barrier created by men, placed on women as no woman has ever passed and graduated the US Army's Rangers training program. To become a US Army Ranger is one of the most physical challenges known to man and is known to be arguably the toughest training in the entire US Armed Forces.

To understand just how incredible the feat that these two women have accomplished is, let's take a close look at the count-less amount men of all walks throughout the history of the mere existence of the Army Rangers, that have fallen short of completing this same exact physical accomplishment and let's not forget the mental strength that had to be involved here.

So to get back to my point discussed earlier, to believe that women in the fitness world can't or aren't capable of accomplishing the same (or similar) physical goals as men, is not only far from being true but a very primitive and incorrect way of thinking period. History has shown us once again that this an out dated way of thinking.

So ladies if you desire your arms to become sexy and fit, let's start by focusing on just that, by saying I can and I will have the arms I so desire. This is all possible with my proper training technique along with proper nutrition.

Equal Opportunity

In the fitness world you can be Oprah Winfrey, Taylor Swift or just an ordinary every day woman, you only get out of training what you put into training. In the fitness world you don't have to have a college degree, nor a huge budget, heck let's be honest you don't even need to have a job to change the way your body looks. Heck, if you really think about it you don't even need weights to change the way you look. Push-ups and sit ups are 100% free and no one can stop you but you. All you really need is what I call the 3D Principals, Dedication, Determination and Discipline.

2. The 3D Principle

The 3D Principal stands for Dedication, Determination and Discipline, this is something I have followed nearly me entire life. I started using it with all my clients years ago in the belief of a person with these principals can accomplish not only their fitness goals but in most all goals they set in life "if" they truly stick to the 3D Principals. I'm a firm believer that when a person decides to make major changes in their life either in fitness or in other aspects, they can better achieve their set goals with the 3D principals.

I have used these three principals in my own fitness goals and have never been disappointed by my end results. By using the these principals I've always known that I've given it my all, 110% and knowing that alone has always made me feel like a winner at the end of the day. Let's discuss what these principals actually are and what they mean to me in the world of fitness.

Dedication

This means to never allow yourself to make any excuses that prevent you from working towards achieving your fitness goals on a daily basis. No matter what the day may bring or how much you may not feel like training. Stay dedicated and train anyway. This includes doing your regular scheduled cardio.

So many times in life we cross paths with people who use phrases like "I'm about to" or "I'm getting ready to. These words are just excuses.

Green Eating & Protein For Leaner Arms
By Daryl BIG"D" Jones

You have to be dedicated to achieve any goal in life no matter if it's growing a leaner set of arms or losing a few unwanted pounds. Dedication has to be a part of your goals in order to be successful. Don't be one of those people who is always about to do this or is getting ready to do that. Be a person who is dedicated to taking action and you'll discover that you'll meet your goals and overcome any roadblocks.

Being dedicated will help propel you to a new level of you. Being dedicated to working out isn't about your short term goals alone, it's about the lifetime rewards you get from pushing yourself hard to create a health benefits that will last a lifetime. So many of us think that training will only make us look better when, in fact, training on a regular basis will also prevent future illnesses and physical decline. In that regard it's very much preventive medicine. It is vitally important to stay focused and dedicated to each realistic physical goal we set - whether it's developing leaner arms or dropping a few unwanted pounds. Dedication is a key player and without it you will surely fall short of your overall fitness and lifestyle goals.

Determination

This will allow you to stay focused and meet the fitness goals you set. You should never quit or give up on anything, such as attempting a lift every day until you achieve it or following your diet to drop those final five pounds. It's so easy to simply give up or quit, as quitting doesn't require any determination.

Green Eating & Protein For Leaner Arms
By Daryl BIG"D" Jones

Quitting can suddenly start to look very appealing as it creates a lot free time to sit around and do nothing. Even worse it allows you to eat unhealthy foods while you sit around and watch other people achieve their goals on television. Quitting sounds so comfortable compared to the hard work that meeting a commitment requires. Determination is what turns quitters into winners so decide right now to stay determined to achieve your fitness goals.

Determination is a mindset, so don't allow your mind to place limits on what's so achievable by not finishing what you started. Setting mental limits will prevent you from achieving the goals you want to go after. You definitely don't want to set mental limits on much leaner you can not only get your arms, but your entire body. Determination will prevent you from being distracted by the negative things people will say when they find out what you want to achieve. Determination will also keep you focused on what you've set your mind to accomplish and allow you to be totally oblivious to anything other than your progress. The power of determination will keep you focused on starting and finishing the goals you set for yourself and allow nothing to divert you from accomplishing them. Mentally implementing determination requires using more powerful internal words such as "I can", and "I will." Determination will push you through the struggles that often occur during your scheduled training sessions and will be your driving force towards meeting your daily workout goals.

Determination will make you successful in both developing a new leaner set of arms and giving you an overall can-do attitude.

Discipline

Discipline is a must in order for us to bring this all together. You have to be disciplined to work toward you fitness goals on a daily basis. Discipline will never allow you to miss your training, or forget to eat your meals on time. Discipline will have you prepare you meals today for tomorrow and discipline will have you stay punctual on, going to the gym on time as well as going to bed on time and getting the much needed rest and for proper recovery.

Discipline plays such an important role in simply dealing with all that life throws at us and we all know life can and most likely will throw us a few curve balls from time to time that's just how life is. But with discipline you can not only get through those curve balls but you can stay focused and make the necessary adjustments to stay on track with the fitness goals that you have set for yourself. Discipline is such a powerful tool to have, discipline will take you to new journeys and new levels in life. Discipline is a must to have in order to achieve the goals you have set for yourself in life, in the gym and out. Discipline will be a huge contributor towards your success, discipline along with your intense determination and dedication will definitely make you stand out from the rest.

Green Eating & Protein For Leaner Arms
By Daryl BIG"D" Jones

Dedication, determination along with discipline will help you achieve your fitness goals with the greatest of ease. You can see how all three of these seem to really say or point to the same direction, and if you truly apply these three principals you will find that in the end of your journey you came out with some pretty successful results in developing your very own set of lean arms. So train hard and train consistently and use the 3D principals and you to will have your very own success story to tell.

MENTAL FOCUS (FIND IT AND FEEL IT)

I personally always tell my clients to find the muscle and feel it. What am I actually saying here? I'm saying to make that mind to muscle connection that we all have subconsciously. Let's take a moment and close our eyes, now make a fist and begin to move your arm up and down as though you were flexing your bicep. Now as you are moving your arm up and down really start to mentally focus on every fiber moving as your arm moves in this upward and downward motion.

This may seem or sound strange right now but as you are becoming more seasoned in your training you will find that by becoming more in tuned with your body you'll be taking your workouts to a totally different level and your training will "feel" explosive. On a lot of sets (not all) I'll close my eyes and get so deeply in tuned with the body part that I'm training, that I'm able to block out the normal level of that burning sensation that we all get, to where I'm able to push past that point giving myself the much needed ability to complete my entire set without the normal signs of fatigue.

Now let's be clear on something here, I'm still feeling the burn the same as anyone else, but with this deep focus I'm able to minimize the burning and push past where most will simply stop. The other benefit of becoming in tuned with your muscles is that you'll be able to create more of what I call, hidden strength, opposed to the person who simply just walks up and grabs a barbell or dumbbell with no mind to muscle connection (no focus at all). Understand that for most this will take time to master and for some depending on your training background you'll discover this technique fairly quickly.

Unfortunately for some of you this connection may never be made, sorry but over the years I'm seen so many try but for whatever reason they just aren't able to make this mind to muscle connection. For those of you who are able to make this connection between your mind and your muscles, this connection will definitely up your game in the gym as well as up your game in your overall training performance. Just be willing to give it a try and be willing to also give it time, as all in this fitness world all things takes time as well as effort. Now go train and find the muscle and feel it.

3. Nutrition

Nutrition for developing lean arms is just as important if not more important as knowing how to properly train them in the gym. You see without proper nutrition you can train your arms or any other body part harder than anyone else in the gym and will have very minimal results if you don't supply the body with the proper nutritional building blocks for change.

Green Eating & Protein For Leaner Arms
By Daryl BIG"D" Jones

There are many different opinions about health and fitness, by many well qualified sources. The problem is that they all truly believe that they're right and all others are wrong. I choose to believe that there are many different approaches in fitness and they "all" work we just need to find the nutritional plan that works best for us as individuals. This is where I differ from the rest I truly believe that is more than one way to get to the other side of the road and particularly when it comes to nutrition and fitness.

Protein

Let's discuss the importance of protein and how it plays a huge role in not only how we look but also in how we feel. Protein is the building blocks for all muscles in our body. Without this main ingredient you'll not only never achieve your muscle changing goals of having lean arms but you'll also be what I often call so many people and that is protein deficient. By being protein deficient your body will always be lose and giggly.

Protein is not only what is needed to grow or develop new muscle on our bodies, but protein also is what keeps us firm, toned and compact. Think of protein like this, the more protein you eat the more additional fat you'll rid your body of. Yes ladies this is true, by not being protein deficient you'll actually lose unwanted fat and start tightening up in areas that were once lose and giggly.

Green Eating & Protein For Leaner Arms
By Daryl BIG"D" Jones

Protein is not only the main building block for obtaining new muscle development but it's also what we need to simply maintain the current muscle on our bodies. Now when I say the word muscle in this instance, I'm not only referring to our visible muscles as in a fitness term, but I'm referring to the muscles we don't visibly see. The muscles in our faces that allow us to smile blink our eyes or to move our mouths as we speak. You see protein keeps us with the muscles we need to simply get around for the day, protein also is the driving nutrient needed to redesign our ordinary arms into a leaner set of arms.

Basic List of Protein

Steak

Turkey

Chicken

Tuna

Fish

Eggs

Protein drinks (low carbohydrates and low fat)

The Carbohydrates

Now when it comes to nutrition and those wanting to shed off a few unwanted pounds, we should shift our focus on what type of carbohydrates we are taking in through-out the day. Unfortunately most focus on the fat intake instead of their carbohydrate intake and that's where many make their biggest mistake. As by now we all know that too many carbohydrates will most definitely place a few un-wanted pounds on us all, especially if we eat the wrong variety of carbohydrates.

Just know that all carbohydrates are "not" created equally. When it comes to carbohydrates let's first focus on what is a carbohydrate? A carbohydrate is everything that isn't a meat item, as there are no carbohydrates in meats. With the exception of processed meats which have tons of sodium and far too many chemicals that's not good for our bodies.

Now let's just think of carbohydrates as being in only two different groups. The first group we will call fibrous carbohydrates which are mainly the color **green** with a couple of exceptions and the second group we will call starchy carbohydrates which are the carbohydrates that provide us with a ton of energy buy unfortunately they also have the potential to put unwanted pounds on a lot of us. Now let's make this even easier for us to distinguish the difference between the two.

Green Eating & Protein For Leaner Arms
By Daryl BIG"D" Jones

Now as I said earlier the fibrous carbohydrates are easy to identify as they're mostly all the color **green** with a few exceptions in the squash family as well as cauliflower & carrots. Although their not green in color they still are in the fibrous family of carbohydrates. Now let's focus on how to identify the starchy carbohydrates. They also are fairly easy to identify as we know already that they are not green in color and that alone helps us tremendously when it comes to identifying which is which.

The starchy carbohydrates are rice, pasta, bread, potatoes, oats, grits, bagels, cereals and so on (I think you get the idea) between the two. The main thing I want you to focus on or realize is that too much or eating too many starchy carbohydrates "will" simply add many unwanted pounds to your body as in fat not muscle. Now as we separate the two carbohydrates please don't think that the starchy carbohydrates don't play a role for the good to our bodies, as they do.

These starchy carbohydrates are an important source of energy for our bodies and also have a good source of nutrients we need such as iron and b vitamins, we just don't ever want to overload on them if watching our weight is part of our fitness goals. Now if you are as I once was, a hard gainer then you'll want to become good friends with the starchy carbohydrates as they will play a significant role in you gaining a little new overall size to your frame.

Fruits vs. Veggies

Now let's start here with an example, we can eat **green** colored veggies all day and get tons of vitamins and nutrients from them without having to worry about getting additional unwanted pounds being placed on our bodies. Now when it comes to eating a fruit or a few fruit baskets (natural carbohydrates full of sugar) we can expect to end up with two different set of results. The bottom line is if you eat too much fruit you'll surely get fat.

You see most people believe just because fruit is naturally grown from the ground that it's ok to eat as much of it as they want. Well fruit is good for you and "yes" it is naturally grown from the ground and yes it does have its place in a healthy diet "but" the problem is that most people simply eat far too much of it which results in gaining unwanted pounds also known as fat. I suggest to people to look at fruit as a dessert instead of a meal, as it's one of nature's greatest treats.

Now when we compare fruits to veggies we can all agree that fruit taste so much better than a bowl of Brussels sprouts, so yes they are our first choice. What we need to keep in mind is that fruit even though it's grown from the ground naturally it still contains one main ingredient that we must not ever over load on and that is sugar. See our bodies don't distinguish the difference from man maid sugar from naturally grown sugar, now here I know many will argue this fact with me and that's ok.

The simple truth is sugar is sugar and it doesn't matter if it's grown from the ground or made in a man maid facility the body will treat all sugars the same. Now let's talk a little more about the benefits of eating a good supply of veggies. Vegetables are an important source of many nutrients, including potassium, fiber, vitamin A, vitamin C and many other daily needed vitamins, which also will aide in our bodies maintaining healthy blood levels as well as keeping our cholesterol levels balanced. Vegetables also assist our digestive tracks, particularly when we're consuming high levels of protein.

When to Eat

Now let's get back to the nutrition needed to re-sculpture our arms, this is really simple. The absolute two most important meals of the day are breakfast to supply your body with the fuel needed to start your day and your after training meal, which you'll need to replenish the body with after an intense training session. Your post training meal should be a healthy well balanced meal packed with (yep you guessed it) protein, protein and more protein. Now let's not only focus on the after training meal, let's also focus and understand that we need to constantly eat throughout the day to supply our bodies with the proper amount of nutrients. In order to have enough protein to properly support the muscle we already have on our bodies, we'll need to break our protein intake down into several meals throughout the day. This is why I love veggies especially asparagus.

Green Eating & Protein For Leaner Arms
By Daryl BIG"D" Jones

Here I'm going against what others recommend doing and that is to only have you consume the amount of protein needed to maintain your "lean" muscle mass. Ladies please also understand that number one you can't tome fat, number two adding a pound of muscle "ISN'T" going to suddenly make you look like a man.

You will become leaner, slimmer, and your natural curves will become even more enhanced. The reason I'm having you do it this way is to maximize your fat loss and to also push your body into a more lean and toned direction. This way of calculating your daily protein intake is a simple fail proof way to not only get your arms leaner look, but this will actually get your entire body to lose unwanted pounds of fat as well.

Please understand that there's no such thing as spot reduction in weight or fat loss. Here's "my" very simple way how to do this. Don't worry about how much body fat you're carrying or how much lean mass you have. Simply take your total body weight and multiply this number by 1. Basically you'll consume 1 gram of protein per pound of your body weight. So let's say you weight 150lbs. then you'll need 150 grams of protein a day. Now let's divide this into 5 meals, which would mean you'll need to have 30 grams of protein with each meal.

Green Eating & Protein For Leaner Arms
By Daryl BIG"D" Jones

Combine any selection of a **green** colored veggie with each serving of protein or with each meal and I assure you that you'll drop a good size of unwanted fat as you are developing your new set of leaner arms.

Example Only (below)
Meal #1 "breakfast" (eat as soon as you can)
Meal #2 (eat 3 hours after meal #1)
Meal #3 "lunch" (eat 3 hours after meal #2)
Meal #4 (eat 3 hours after meal #3)
Meal #5 "dinner" (eat 3 hours after meal #4)

Most of you may be say I have to eat 5 meals a day? This will make me fat gain more weight "and" in unwanted places. Well the truth is that you'll actually lose more weight and fat by eating more frequently throughout the day. Let me explain how this works.

Imagine sitting at a red light in your car, you have your foot on the brake and your engine is at an idle speed, meaning the motor of your car is at a relaxed speed burning less fuel. Now when the light turns green you'll take your foot off the brake and you'll now press down on the accelerator and the motor will now begin to come out of the relaxed state it was in and it will now speed up now more fuel is being burned in the process.

Green Eating & Protein For Leaner Arms
By Daryl BIG"D" Jones

Well this is the is the exact same way our bodies and our metabolisms respond when we go from eating one or two meals a day to suddenly eating every 3 hours. The more frequently we eat the more our motors (our metabolisms) speeds up to burning more fat off our bodies. So in short the more "frequently" you eat the faster you'll speed up your metabolism. Now let's go back to why I want you to consume 1 gram of protein per pound of your total body weight. The truth is that you can actually consume "less" protein than I asked you to do and still get some awesome results.

Again the reason "I" ask you to use my method so you'll have phenomenal changes in your overall physique not just in your arms. Always remember the more protein you eat the more compact, lean and toned you'll become. Simply put the more protein you eat the more fat you'll lose. So rule number one is that immediately after training you want to eat as soon as possible (ASAP) why? Because after you have trained your arms really hard you'll need to help them change into a leaner more toned arm by supplying them with recovery food/nutrients needed.

Helpful Tips

Now a few things on salad dressing that most people "don't" know!!! Now when you purchase a fat free salad dressing please understand that it is 'ONLY" fat free up to the serving limit also known as per serving listed on the item. So for example if it says FAT FREE and the serving size is 3 table spoons well guess what? If you go beyond that serving size listed, it is NO LONGER FAT FREE!!!

So a fat free salad dressing is fine just DO NOT use more than the serving size listed OK! Now let's talk about green vegetables the awesome thing about when we eat green colored veggies is that we can eat them all day everyday in any amounts we want and they will "NEVER" store as fat "smile" it is impossible for them to be stored as fat no matter how much we eat nor does it matter what time we eat them. This is why I never got into just how much of them to eat. Just remember again when you feel full "STOP" eating and always make sure to consume your protein first before you get full. Our **green** colored veggies are also an excellent source of fiber, so eat up!!!

Important

Eat on time (every 3 hours) always eat your protein before you become full, so if or when you become full you've already consumed the most important nutrient on your plate or bowl. Next I want you to "STOP" eating when you become full no matter what's remaining on your plate or bowl. If this occurs often you'll simply need to readjust your serving sizes the next day to prevent wasting of food.

Make every meal with a good serving of protein and any **green** colored veggie and remember veggies won't make you fat so never go hungry.

Green colored veggies are packed with nutrients as well as a good supply of fiber, which is definitely needed to move the consumption of protein properly throughout the body. Ok these are simple helpful tips that I again put together for "all" my clients, I truly hope they become helpful to you as well.

Water Intake

Last but not least you'll need to consume a minimum of 1 ounce of water per pound of your body weight, broken down into 6-8 sections of water a day, as the proper intake of water will be needed to make your arms grow. Let's discuss the importance of drinking water a bit further than simply aiding in our sexy lean arm program. Drinking the right amount of water will vary from person to person as we all weigh different amounts.

For example if you're a person who weighs 120lbs then you'll need 120 ounces of water a day and if you're a person (like myself) who weight 250lbs then I'll need to drink 250 ounces of water a day, but what won't vary is the need for us all to drink enough water every single day, no matter what your goals are in fitness or in simply being a healthy person.

Green Eating & Protein For Leaner Arms
By Daryl BIG"D" Jones

Water has many health benefits to us all, and since our bodies are made up of about 60% of actual water, drinking enough on a daily basis helps maintains the body's fluids balance. Water also aides in the transporting of nutrients throughout the body, and it helps to regulate the bodies temperature as well as allows our bodies to properly digest our foods. As you can see water has so many health benefits to us, far more than what most us may have initially first thought.

If that doesn't motivate you to want to keep track of your water intake and to make sure that you drink enough water throughout the day maybe this will, water also helps significantly with weight loss. Many studies over the years have shown that drinking enough water will aide in weight loss, as in helping shed a few unwanted pounds off. Drinking water will simply make you feel as though you're full and will assist those of you who want to lose a few unwanted pounds find it easier to consume less calories than you normally would.

Drinking plenty of water also keeps our kidneys healthier, gives us energy, helps maintain or develop a healthier looking skin, and my own favorite reason for drinking water is that not only will your body be healthier but your muscles will look fuller and you'll be stronger in the gym, so please drink water if you truly are wanting to have lean and well toned arms and if you simply want to live longer.

Experiences

I've gotten my mind opening theories from being a guy who competed for many years as a bodybuilder and from seeing unbelievable size muscle back stage. I spoke to countless former competitors and listened to what they did to achieve their new muscle development. I also shared my own techniques with them as to exactly what I did to change the look of my own physique. In the mist of doing all that I tried almost every program there is to get bigger muscles on a leaner body and in my journey I came up with my very own program that I felt helped me the most and that I feel will also help you as well.

4. Workout

Skull crushers
Standing barbell curls
Cable press downs (straight bar)
Dumbbell hammer curls
Body weight dips
Side laterals

TRICEPS (EXERCISE #1)
Skull Crushers

Now let's start training and let's begin with the all to famous skull crushers also known as kick-outs and let's load it with a fairly controllable weight using a straight bar. Make sure that you don't load this up with a over challenging weight as we will be doing 4 set of 25 repetitions for our triceps (the upper back part of the arm) with very little rest in between each set.

The goal is to perform the first set of 25 repetitions and take a short rest of 60 seconds. Then immediately begin the second set of 25 repetitions and repeat the 60 seconds of rest. Then begin set number three and repeat until you have successfully completed all four sets of 25 repetitions, equaling a total of 100 repetitions.

Green Eating & Protein For Leaner Arms
By Daryl BIG"D" Jones

Now the reality is that most of you will need to stop and rest in the middle of the set. This is normal until you get your body conditioned to a higher level and then you'll be able to conduct all four sets with stopping any longer than the 60 seconds specified in between each set. For those who do need to rest in the middle of the 25 repetition set, try not to rest for longer than 15-30 seconds and resume where you left off at in your count, until you reach 25 repetitions.

TRICEPS (EXERCISE #1)
Skull Crushers 4 set's of 25 repetitions
100 repetitions total.

Grip the bar with thumbs on top.

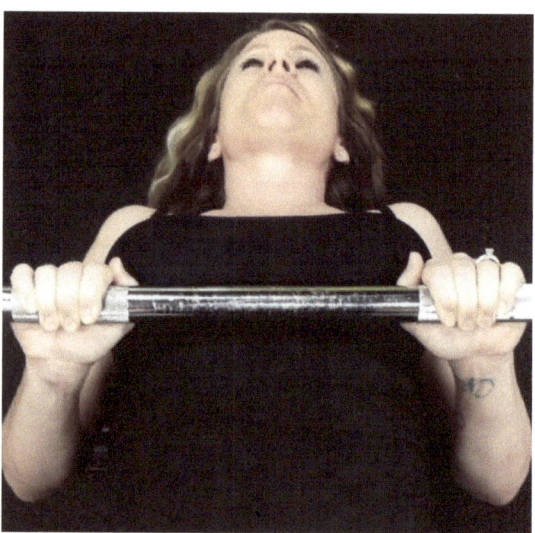

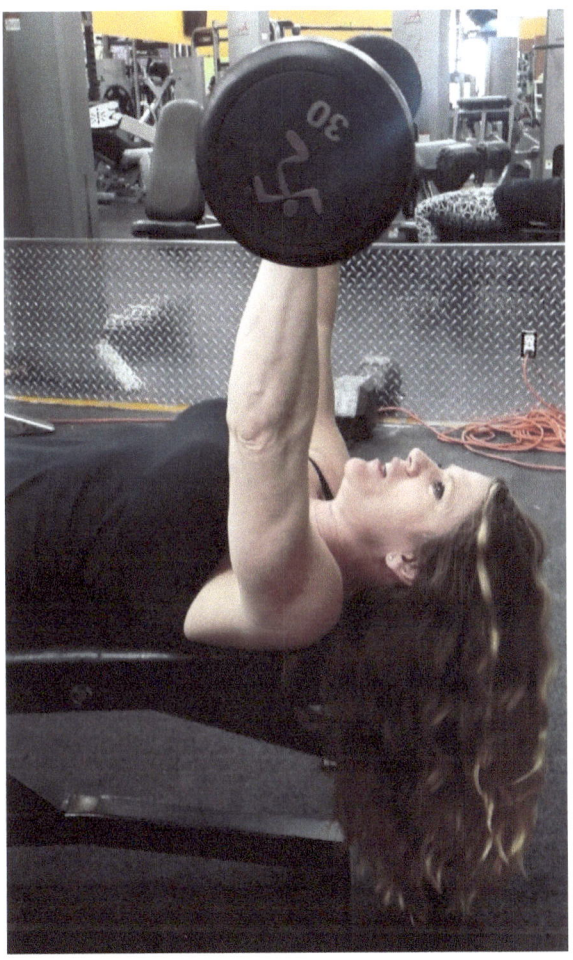

At the top of this movement, begin to inhale just before bringing the weight downward.

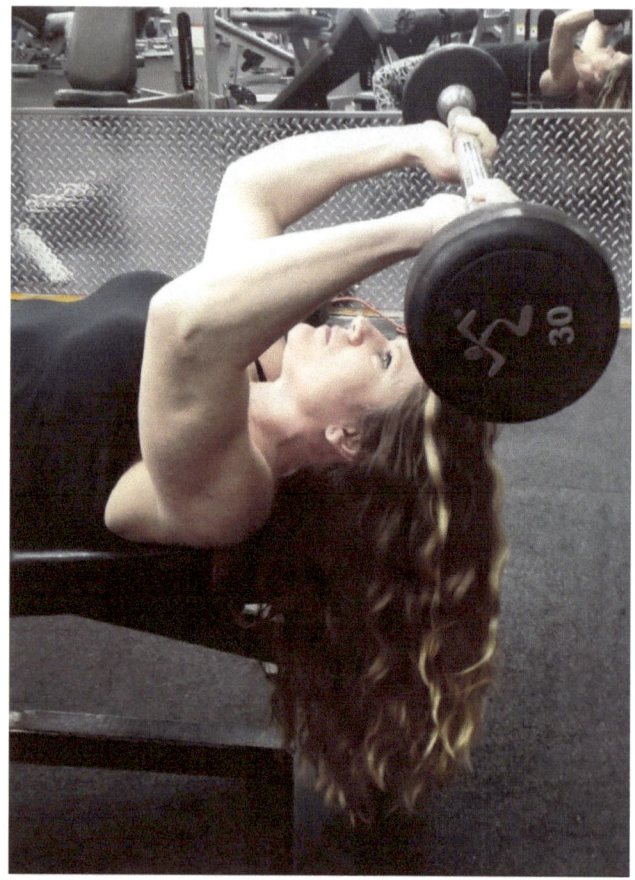

Continue inhaling as you're bringing the weight downward. Also keep a tight hand grip on the bar, as this will give you more power as you're performing this movement.

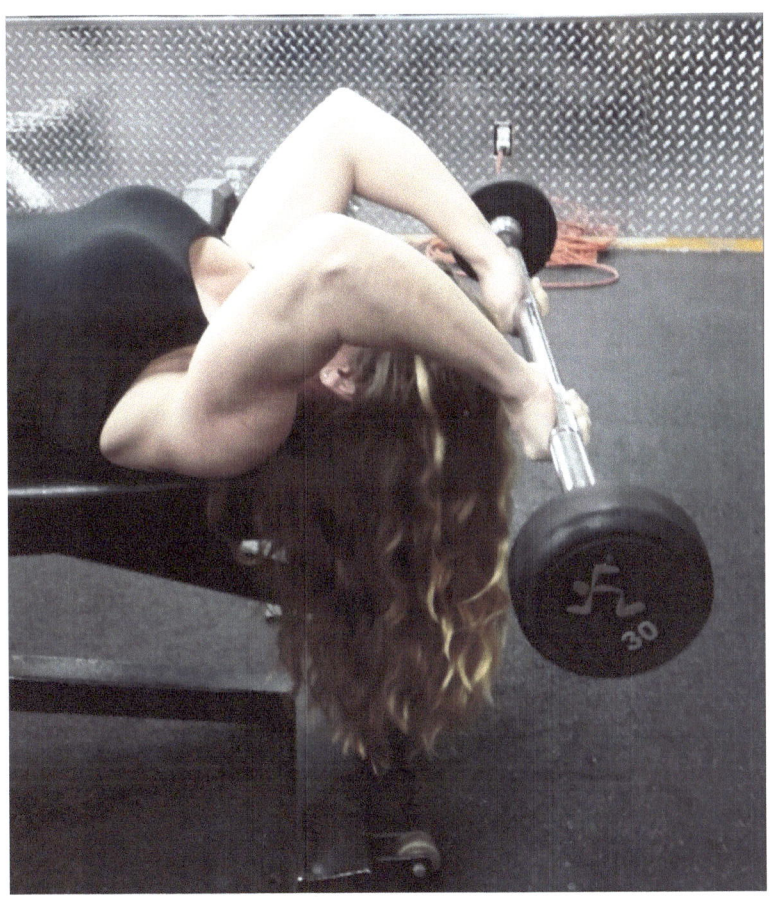

Now just before powering the weight upward begin to exhale, but don't fully exhale until you are at the top/completion of the repetition.

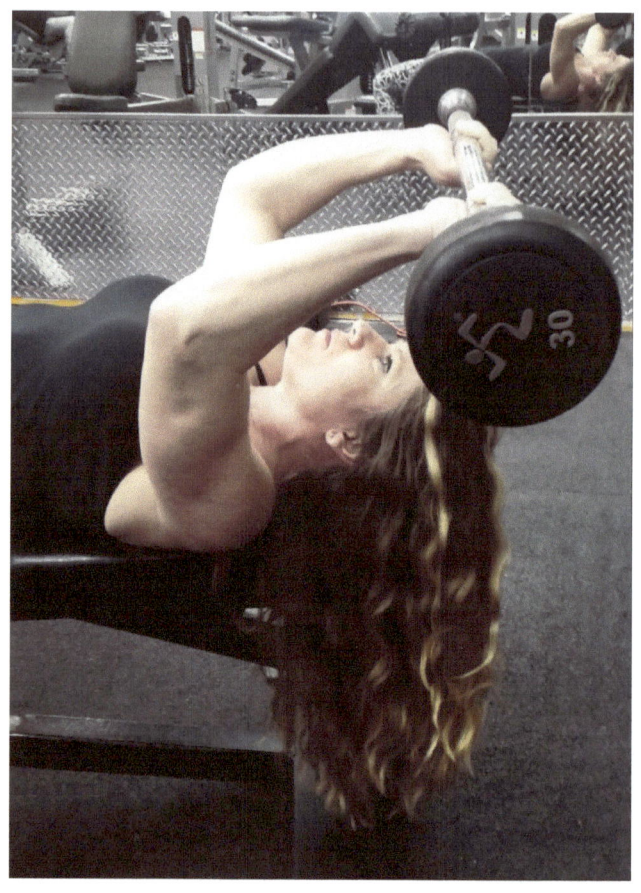

Continue to blow out (exhaling) as you are bringing the weight back upward.

Green Eating & Protein For Leaner Arms
By Daryl BIG"D" Jones

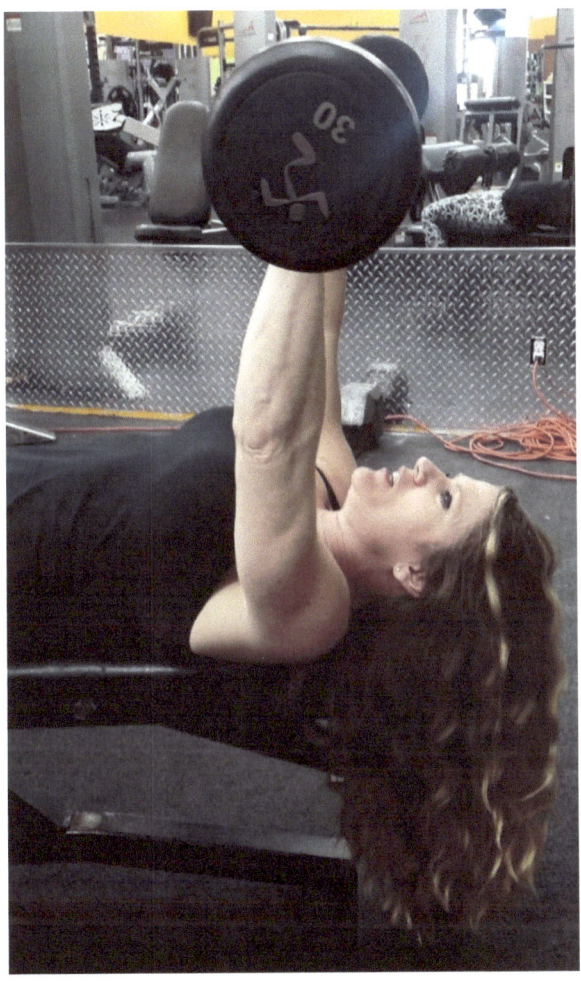

As you return to the top of this movement fully exhale and repeat for 25 reps for 4 sets, 100 reps in total. Remember to only rest for 60 seconds in between each set.

Standing Barbell Curls

Now that our triceps are full of blood with a good pump, let's now focus on our biceps with a traditional straight bar standing barbell curl, using a standard shoulder width grip. Select a weight that you know is light weight enough for you complete 25 repetitions straight for 4 sets, making your total count, 100 repetitions, just as we did above with the skull crushers.

Remember try your best not to rest for longer than 60 seconds between sets. This will be tough but you can do it. If you start to tire do as many as you can and split the reps if needed into repetitions of 5 for example if you are rep 10 and you decide you need to rest, don't set the weight down "but" take a breather and then make a 5 rep commitment and go for 15 reps and so on, until you complete the entire 25 repetitions. Ok we're not done with our training yet so let's get back to training.

Standard hand grip.

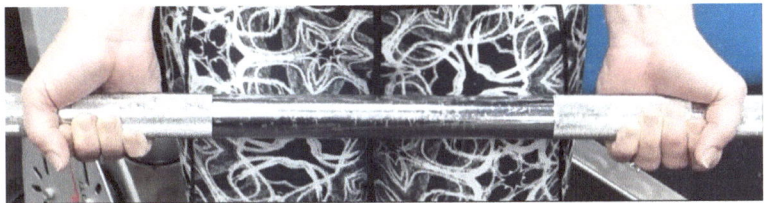

Here we'll use a traditional standard hand grip as we perform the standing barbell curl. By gripping the bar tightly you may find that you will discover additional strength to perform this exercise. We also will want to focus on correct breathing patterns, which will be explained in the photos below each illustrated photo. Breathing properly will definitely maximize your ability to complete each set of 25 repetitions, just as improper breathing will definitely hinder your full potential in performing this exercise.

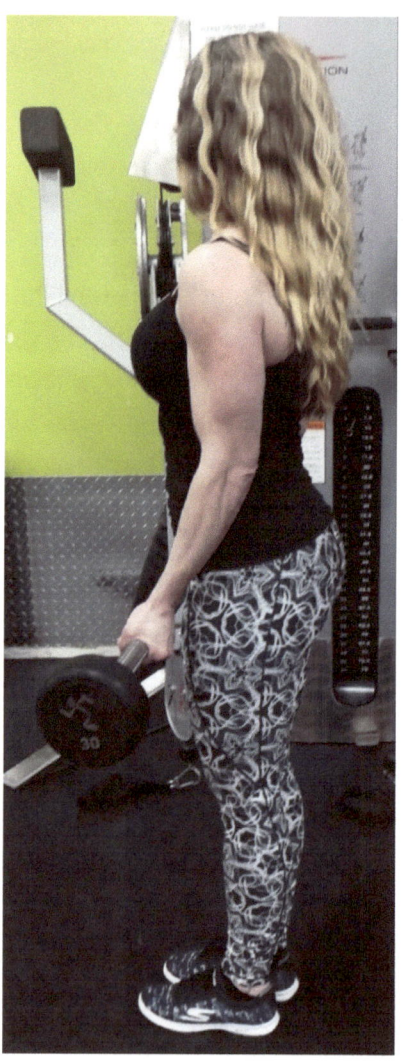

Take a deep breath, filling up your lungs and just before curling upward begin to exhale.

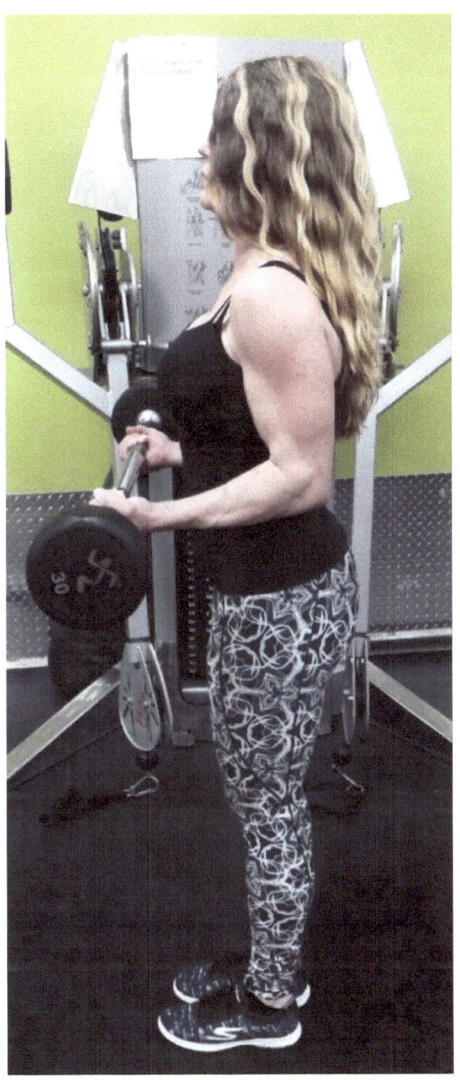

Continue to blow out (exhaling) as you are curling the weight upward.

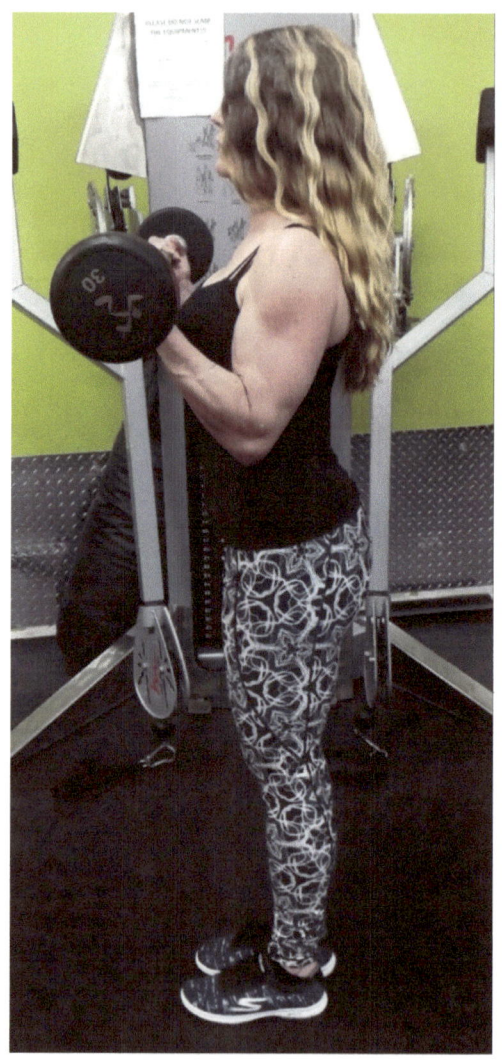

Now fully exhale at the top and repeat for 25 reps. Do 4 sets of 25reps for a total of 100 repetitions.

Cable Press Downs

Now let's return back to our triceps and let's now do another 4 sets of 25 repetitions with the exact same rest periods as above 60 second in between if training alone and if training with a workout partner rest only while your training partner is performing their set of 25 reps. By now I'm sure at this point you can see the importance of your mind being set for achievement as this is going to a game of mental strength as well as physical strength.

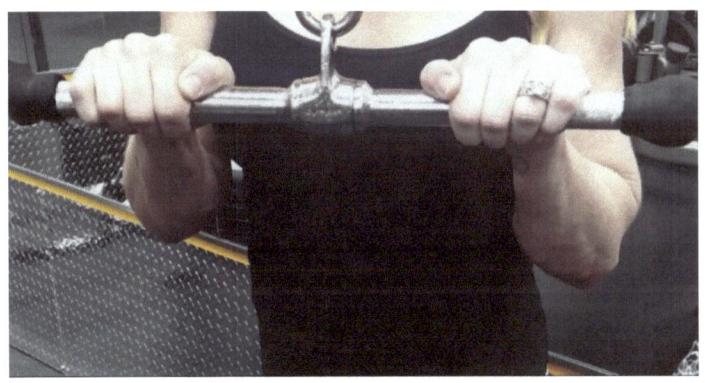

Thumbs on top.

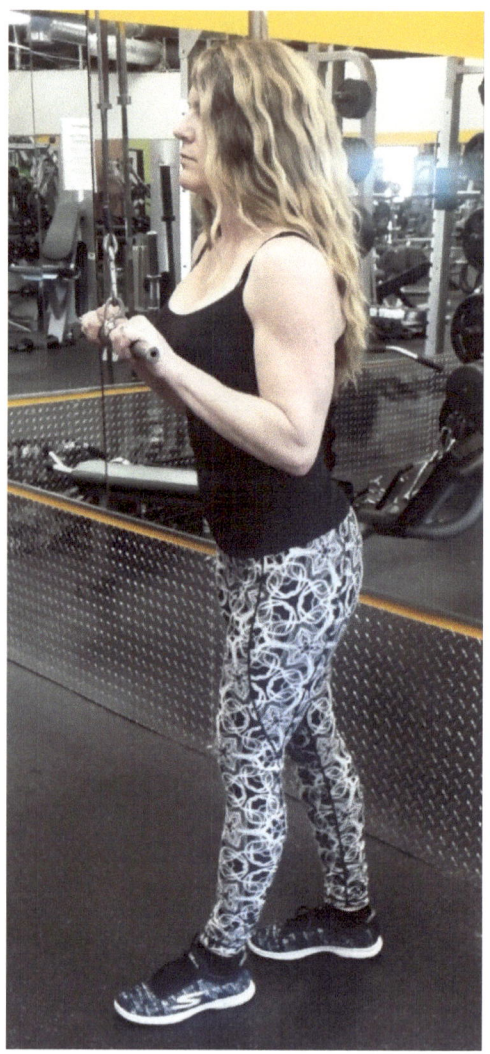

Lean slightly inward towards the cable, take a deep breath (side view) and just before pressing downward, begin to exhale.

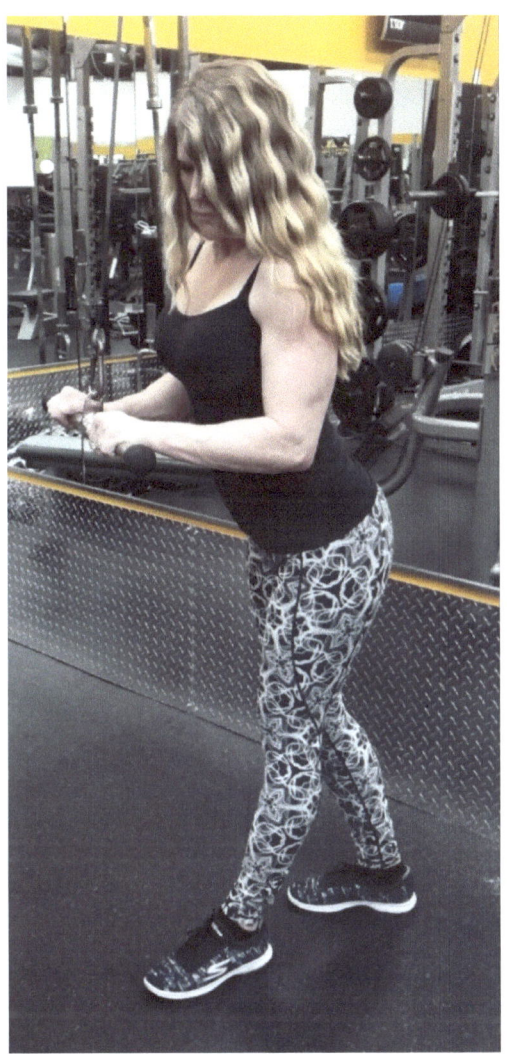

Continue exhaling (blowing out) as you're pressing the cable straight bar downward.

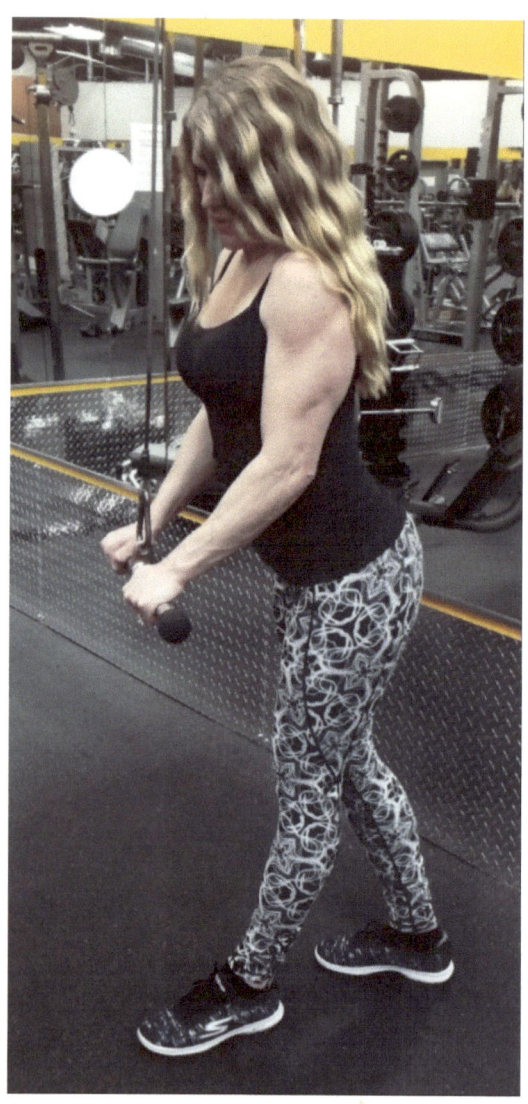

¾ of the way down still exhaling (blowing out) as you're pressing downward.

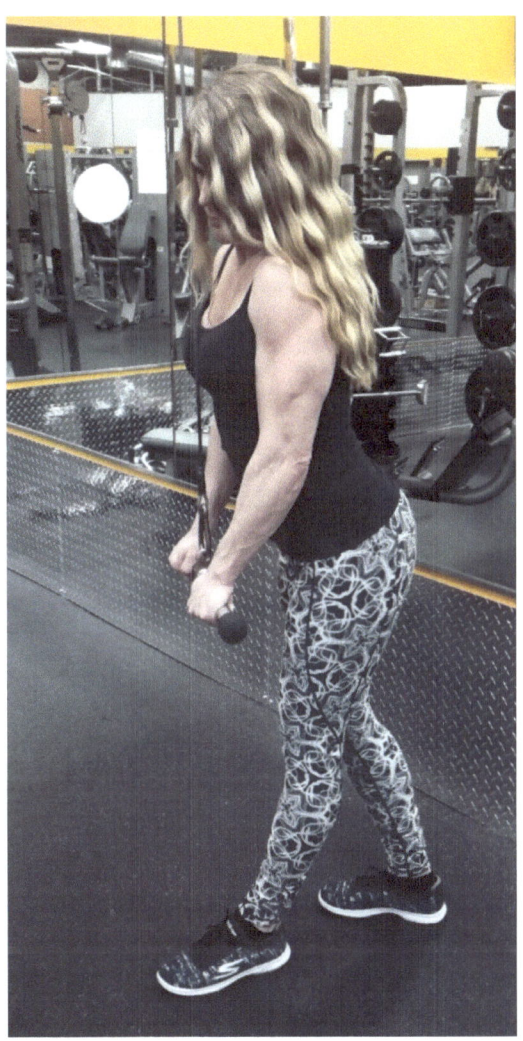

Fully exhale at the bottom and begin inhaling as you're returning to the original start position and repeat.

Dumbbell Hammer Curls

Now let's return for one more set of biceps and let's do a set of dumbbell hammer curls standing or sitting the choice is yours, and let's do another 4 sets of 25 reps for a total of 100 repetitions. Again only take a 60 second rest between sets unless you are training with a workout partner. Then only rest while they perform their set of 25 reps. Make each set of 25 repetitions a challenge.

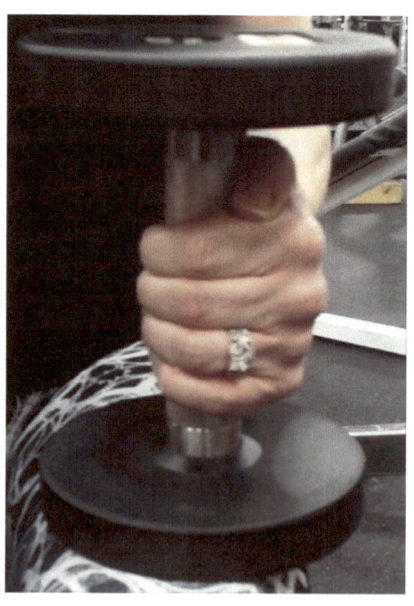

Hammer Curls Hand Position

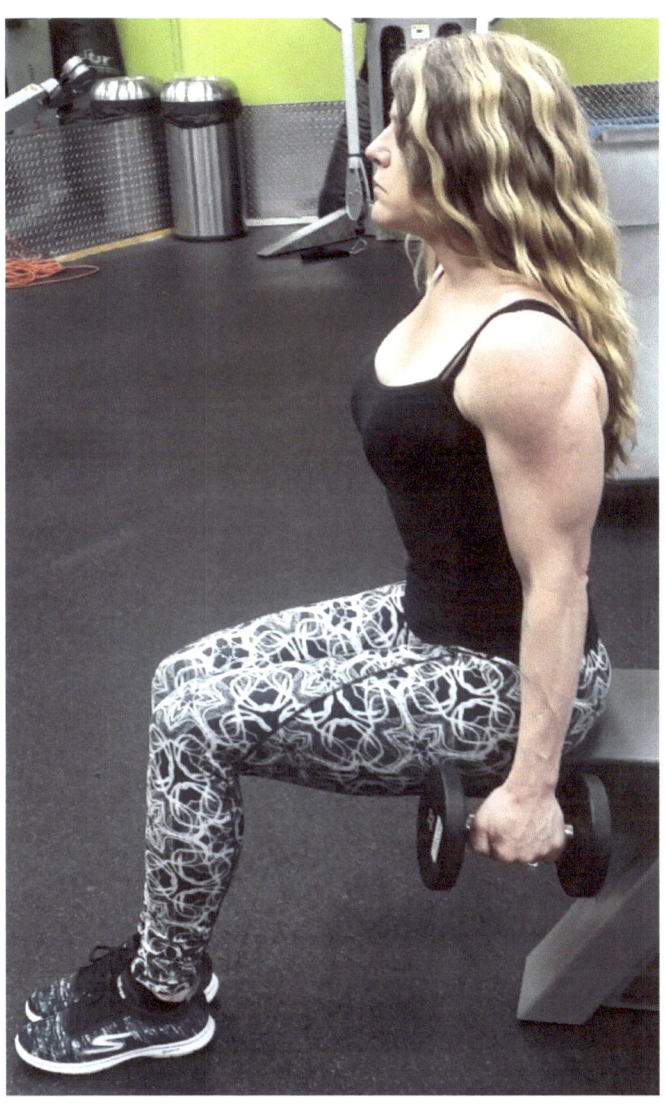

**Take a deep breath and just before curling
upward begin to slowly blow out.**

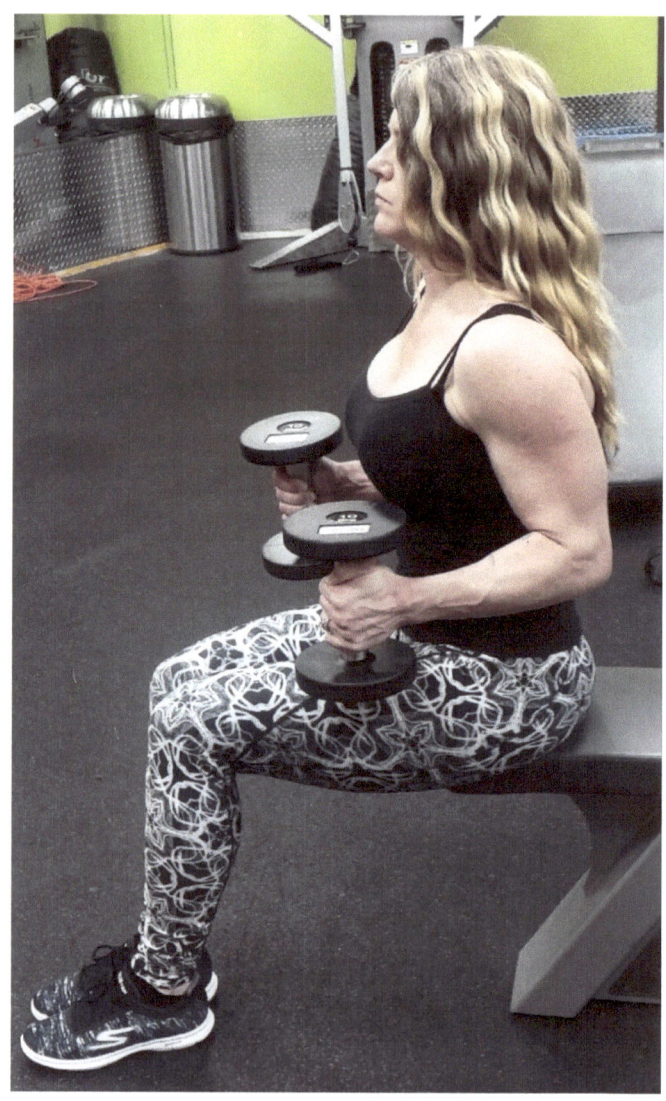

Continue blowing outward as you're curling the weight upward.

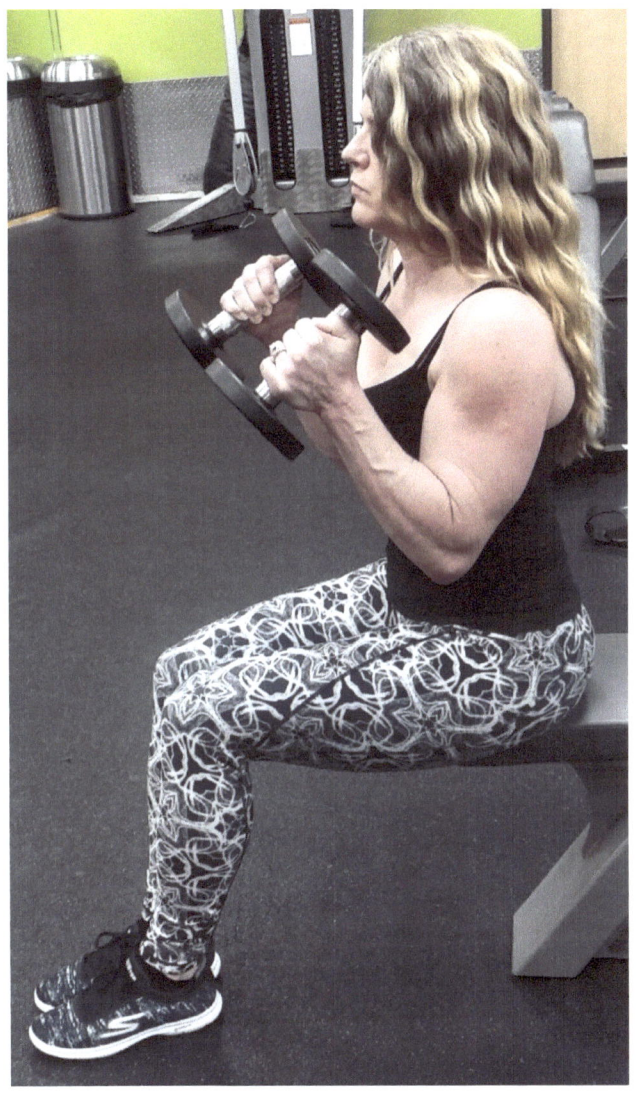

Fully exhale at the top of the movement and repeat. Do 4 sets of 25 reps for a total of 100 reps.

Body Weight Dips

Now for the final exercise of the day, we will move to body weight dips, here we will also do another 4 sets of 25 reps for a total of 100 repetitions. Make sure that at the bottom of each repetition we are going deep enough to really stress the triceps (backside of the upper arm) for change.

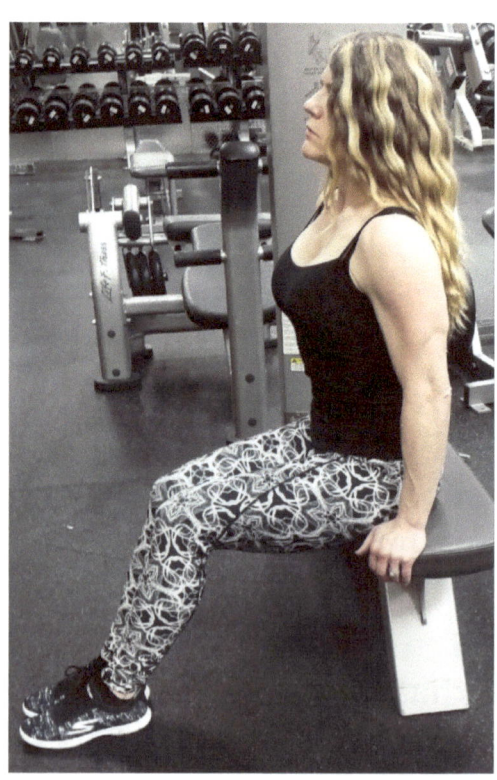

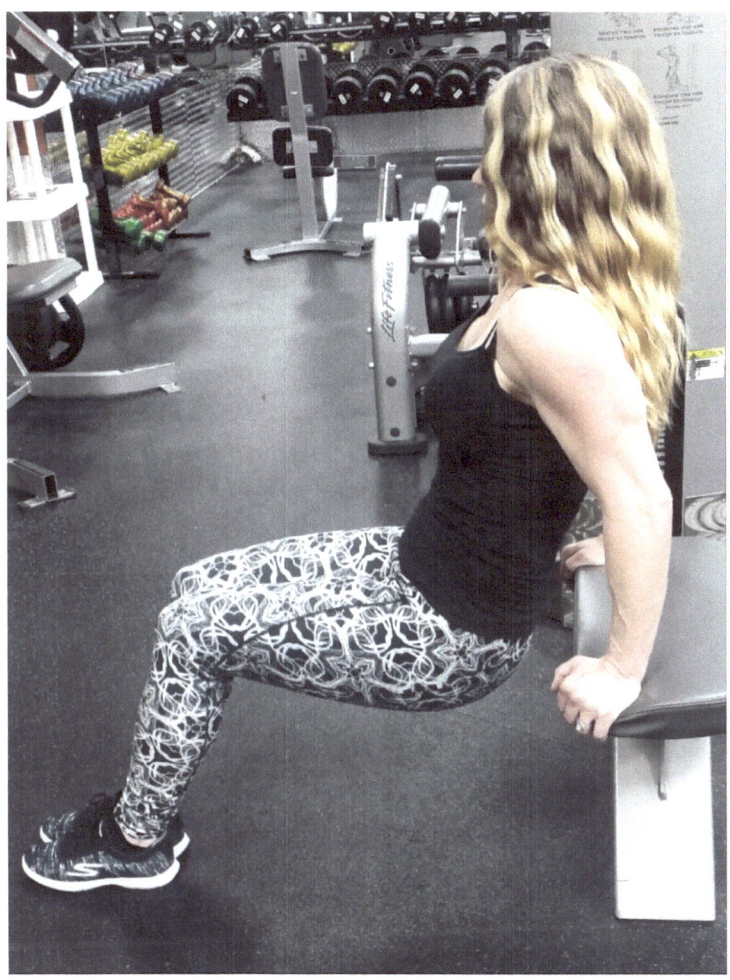

At the start position (shown above) begin to inhale as you are lowering yourself downward.

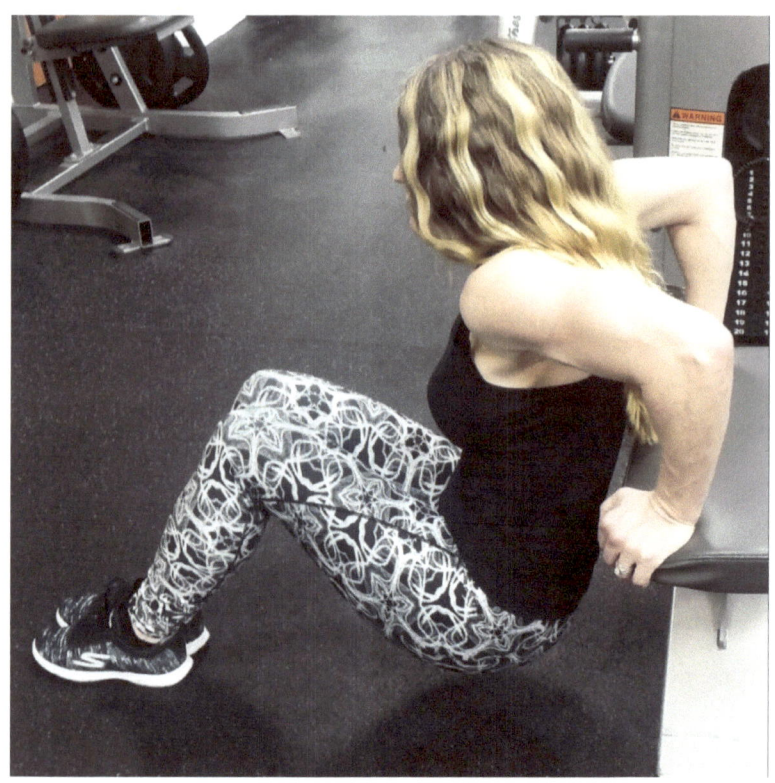

Continue to inhale as you are lowering your body downward.

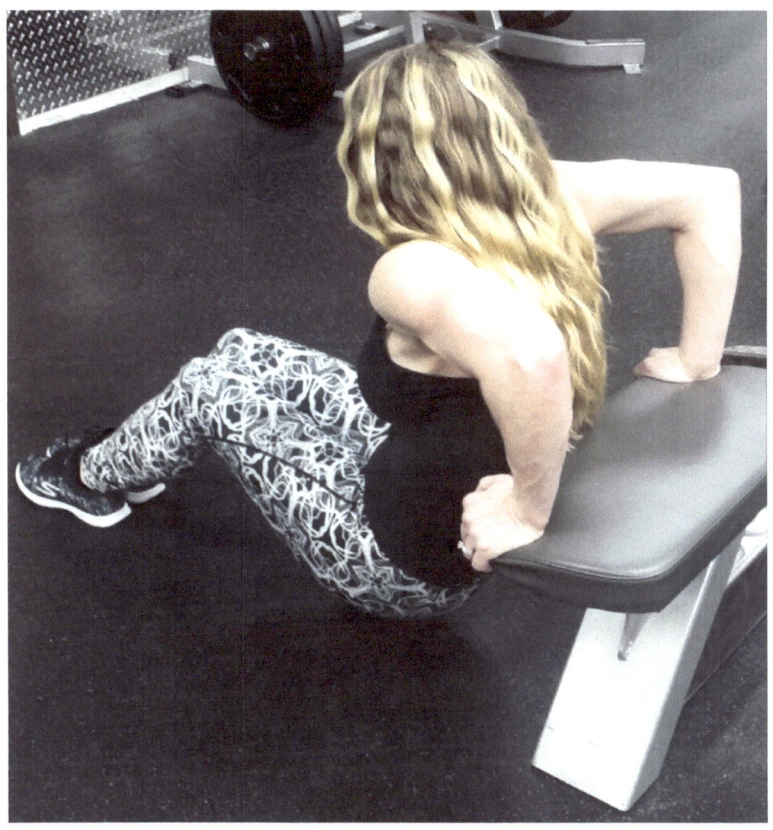

Now begin to blow out (exhale) as you are now beginning to press your body upward. Notice how the shoulder has dropped slightly below the elbow.

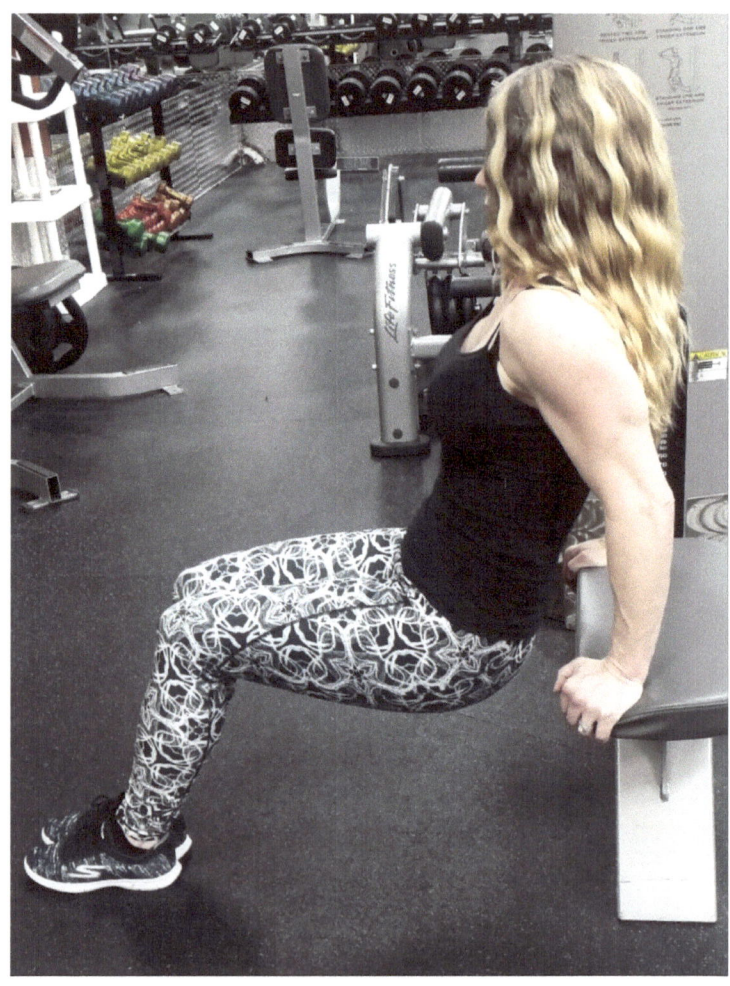

Fully exhale at the "top" of the movement and begin inhaling just before beginning the downward movement again.

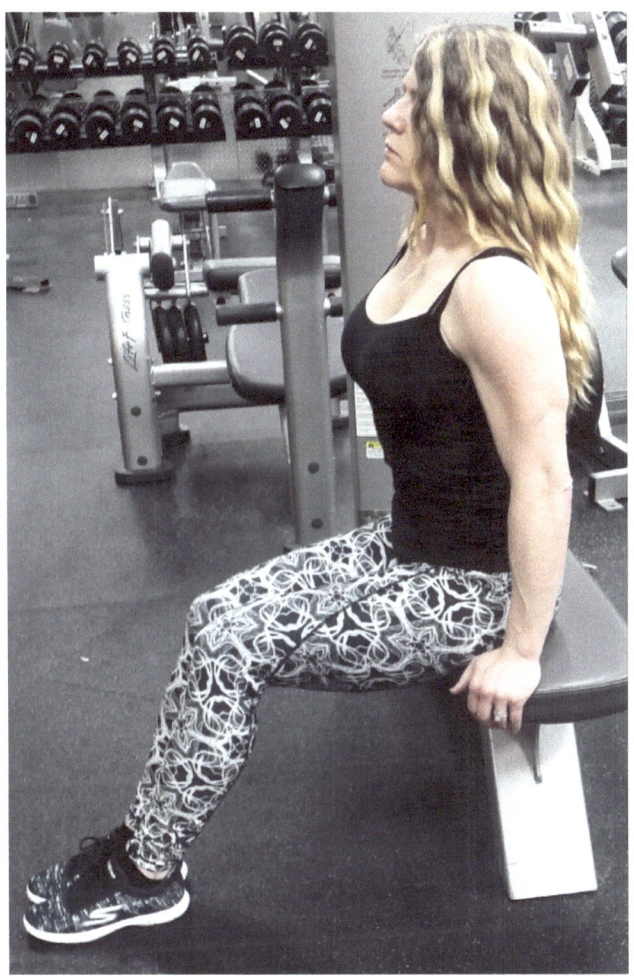

Do 4 sets of 25 repetitions for a total of 100 repetitions. Make sure to rest for "only" 60 seconds in between each set.

Side Laterals

We will now do side laterals as the final exercise towards developing sexy fit arms. Side laterals are a shoulder (Side Deltoid) exercise that will change the look of any arm when performed correctly on a regular basis. This is an exercise that will separate the shoulders and arms with a nice athletic detailed cut. This exercise alone will help get rid of what I call a "SHARM" you may be asking yourself what the heck is a "SHARM" it's when a person has a shoulder and arm smoothly blended together into one long looking muscle. This lack of definition alone will destroy the potential look of an awesome set of arms. This separation looks great on a woman and will simply enhance the overall appearance of a nice set of "sexy" arms. So as all the above exercises we will be doing 4 sets of 25 repetitions for a total of 100 repetitions. Make sure to do your best and only rest for no longer than 60 seconds in between each set. Ladies you "can" do this.

NOTE: You can do this without any weights until you get stronger for additional resistance.

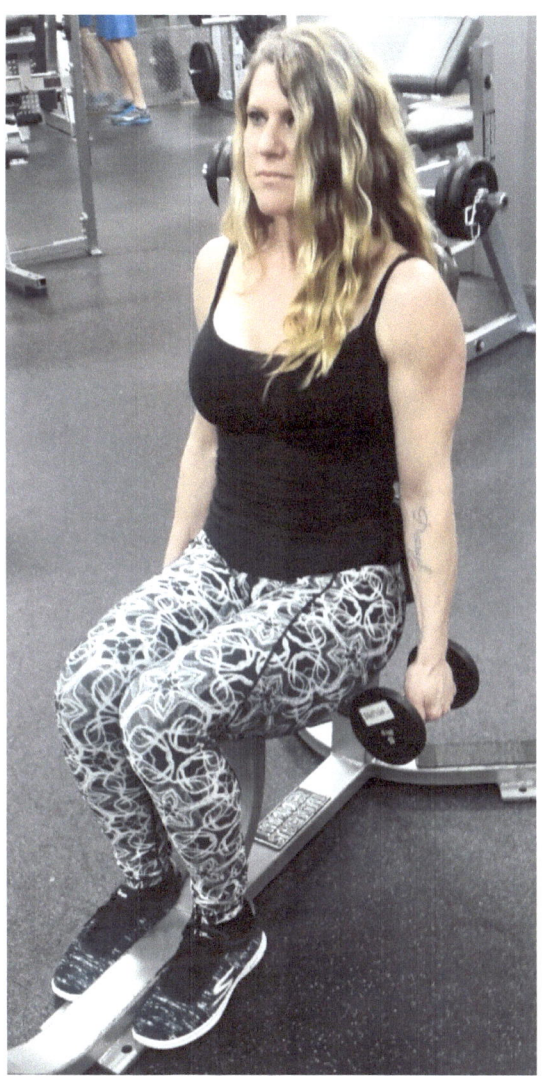

Starting position, take a deep breath before beginning the upward movement.

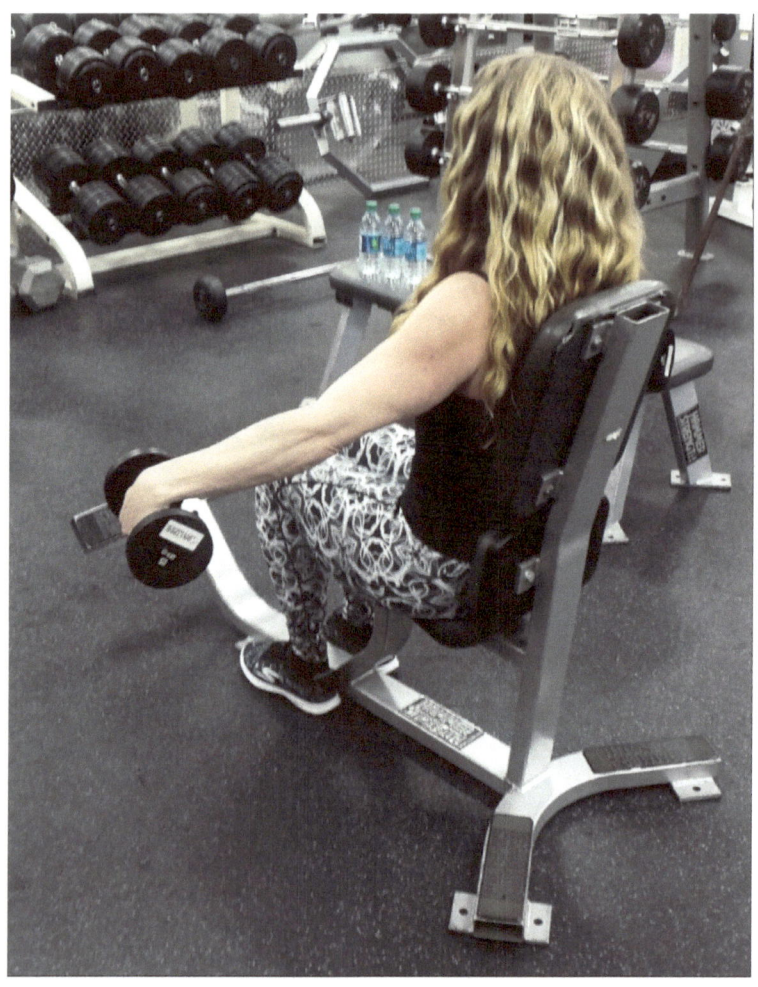

Exhale as you begin to lift upward. Lift up with a "wide" outward left to right reach, keeping the arms straight but without locking the joints. Keep a slight bend in the elbow.

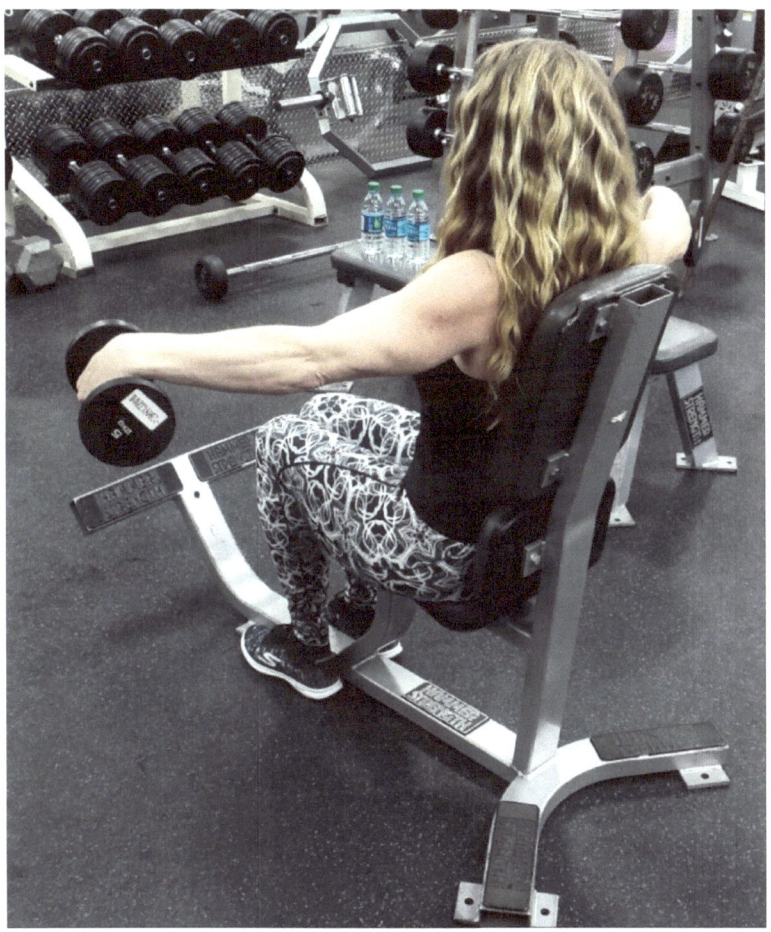

Continue to exhale as you are bringing the weights upward. Notice how the hands and wrist are bent downward, gripping the dumbbells in a hooking fashion.

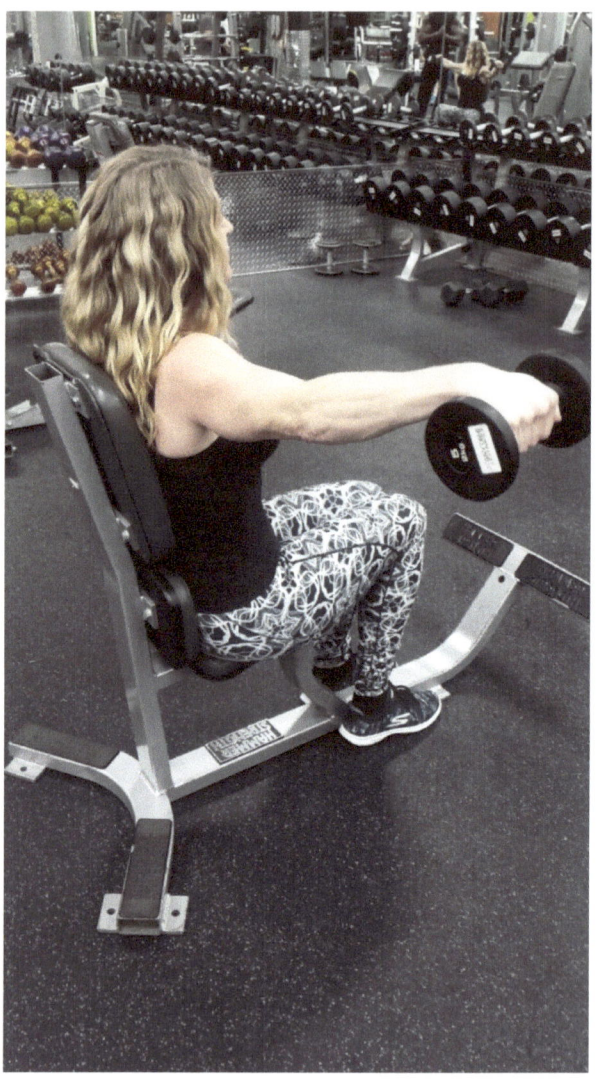

Here as we are now at the top of the movement, you'll notice how the elbow has come up equally as high as the shoulder.

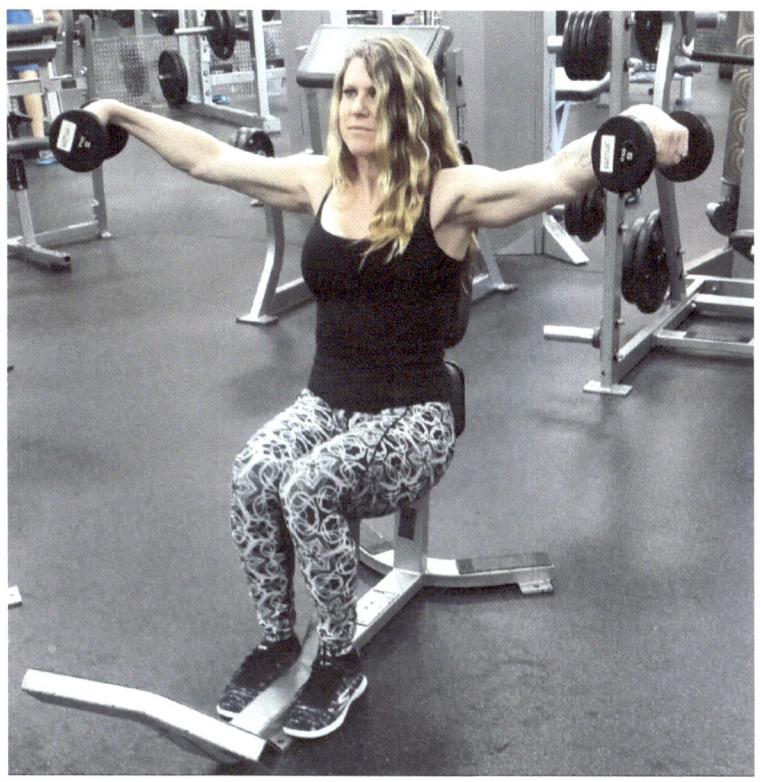

Fully exhale at the top of this movement and as you are now about to lower the arms in a controlled fashion, begin to inhale as the weight is being lowered. Again notice the bend in the wrist and the level of the elbow raising upward as high the shoulders themselves.

OBSTACLES

Expect things to not go perfectly and don't get depressed or lose motivation simply because something unexpected happens. Always focus on the positive and don't brood on the negatives. You can overcome obstacles with some of these ideas:

If you miss a training day, simply start where you left off the very next day.

If you miss a scheduled meal don't eat two meals on the next scheduled eating time simply eat the next meal and go on from there.

If your time is limited beyond your normal control, don't miss the entire.

Workout, simply go into the gym and train with the available time you have (don't miss the entire training if possible).

These simple approaches that should aide you in successfully achieving your fitness goals, just know none of us are perfect but try to always give 110% effort toward your goals and I'm absolutely sure you'll be happy with your final results.

Train Hard and Then Train Harder!

You now have all the tools you need to develop your own set of head-turning lean arms. So now it's time to get in the gym and train hard – and after that, as I always say, then train even harder!

www.ingramcontent.com/pod-product-compliance
Lightning Source LLC
Chambersburg PA
CBHW050816290526
45792CB00001B/138